Allergic Rhinitis Demystified

Holistic Methods to Treat Allergies, End Inflammation, and Restore Respiratory Health

(Things You Must Know)

By

Isabella White

Table of Contents

Introduction

Allergic rhinitis is a condition that occurs when the immune system overreacts to certain substances in the air, called allergens, that are usually harmless to most people. These allergens can trigger inflammation and irritation in the nose, eyes, throat, and sinuses, leading to sneezing, a runny nose, itchy eyes, and nasal congestion.

Allergic rhinitis can affect the affected person's quality of life, sleep, and productivity. It may also increase the risk of developing other conditions, such as asthma, sinusitis, and ear infections. Different types of allergic rhinitis exist, depending on the frequency, severity, and triggers. The main types are:

- **Seasonal allergic rhinitis,** also known as hay fever, occurs during certain times of the year, usually spring, summer, or fall when the pollen levels from trees, grasses, and weeds are high. This allergic rhinitis affects about 8% of adults and 9% of children in the United States.

- **Perennial allergic rhinitis** occurs year-round and is usually caused by indoor allergens such as dust mites, animal dander, cockroaches, and mold spores. This allergic rhinitis affects about 10% of adults and 13% of children in the United States.

- **Occupational allergic rhinitis** is triggered by exposure to allergens or irritants in the workplace, such as wood dust, flour, latex, chemicals, or animal proteins. This type of allergic rhinitis can affect people who work in various occupations, such as bakers, farmers, veterinarians, cleaners, and health care workers.

Difference Between Allergic and Non-Allergic Rhinitis

Allergic rhinitis and non-allergic rhinitis are two types of rhinitis, which is a condition that causes inflammation and irritation in the nose, eyes, throat, and sinuses. The main difference between them is the cause of the symptoms. Allergic rhinitis is caused by the immune system overreacting to certain substances in the air, called allergens, that are usually harmless to most people. Non-allergic rhinitis is not caused by allergies but by other factors that trigger swelling in the lining of the nose, such as irritants, weather, infections, foods, drinks, hormones, or medications.

Some common symptoms of both types of rhinitis are sneezing, a runny nose, nasal congestion, and mucus in the throat. However, allergic rhinitis often also causes itchy noses, eyes, and throats, which are not typical of non-allergic rhinitis. Allergic rhinitis may be seasonal, perennial, or occupational, depending on the symptoms' frequency, severity, and triggers. Non-allergic rhinitis can be acute or chronic and may have various subtypes, such as vasomotor, atrophic, gustatory, or exercise-induced rhinitis.

Diagnosing allergic and non-allergic rhinitis is based on a comprehensive history and physical examination, and sometimes also on allergy testing, such as skin or blood tests. The treatment of rhinitis depends on the symptoms' type, cause, and severity. It may include antihistamines, nasal corticosteroids, decongestants, leukotriene modifiers, allergen avoidance, immunotherapy, or surgery.

The Impact of Allergic Rhinitis on Physical and Mental Health

Allergic rhinitis is not just a nuisance that causes nasal symptoms such as sneezing, runny nose, and congestion. It can also significantly impact the physical and mental health of the affected person, affecting their quality of life, sleep, productivity, and mood. Some of the physical effects of allergic rhinitis are:

- Increased risk of developing other conditions, such as asthma, sinusitis, ear infections, and oral allergy syndrome.
- An impaired sense of smell and taste can affect appetite and nutrition.
- Reduced exercise tolerance and physical activity can lead to weight gain and cardiovascular problems.

- Poor sleep quality and quantity can cause daytime fatigue, impaired memory, and reduced alertness.

Some of the mental effects of allergic rhinitis are:

- Increased levels of stress, anxiety, and depression may be related to the inflammatory response, the social stigma, or the reduced self-esteem associated with the condition.
- Decreased cognitive performance and academic achievement may be due to the distraction, medication side effects, or sleep deprivation caused by the condition.
- Seasonal variation, hormonal changes, or the chronic nature of the condition may influence lowered mood and emotional well-being.
- As you can see, allergic rhinitis can have a profound impact on your physical and mental health and should not be ignored or underestimated.

The Purpose and Benefits of this Book

This book aims to provide you with holistic, natural, and effective strategies to overcome allergic rhinitis. This condition affects millions of people worldwide and can harm your physical and mental health. By reading this book, you will learn:

- What allergic rhinitis is, what causes it, and how it can be diagnosed and treated.
- How to identify and avoid the allergens that trigger your symptoms and reduce your exposure to them.
- How to use natural remedies, such as herbs, supplements, essential oils, and homeopathy, to relieve your symptoms and boost your immune system.
- Learn how to improve respiratory health through adopting a healthy lifestyle, including diet, exercise, stress management, and sleep hygiene, to prevent and control inflammation.
- Learn how to manage the emotional and social challenges of living with allergic rhinitis and improve your well-being.

This book is based on the latest scientific research and the author's personal and professional experience. Following the holistic methods in this book, you can treat your allergies, end inflammation, and restore your respiratory health without relying on medications that may have side effects or lose effectiveness over time. You will also be able to improve your quality of life, sleep, productivity, and mood and enjoy a happier and healthier life.

Chapter 1

The Holistic Approach to Allergic Rhinitis

What is Holistic Medicine, and How Does it Differ from Conventional Medicine?

Holistic medicine is a type of healing that focuses on the entire person, considering their body, mind, spirit, and emotions to achieve optimal health and wellness. It employs different healthcare practices, from conventional to alternative, to treat an individual.

The belief behind holistic medicine is that a person's physical, mental, spiritual, and social aspects are interconnected, and any imbalance in one aspect can lead to illness. Therefore, the primary goal of this form of medicine is to maintain balance.

Conventional medicine, also called Western medicine or modern medicine, is when healthcare professionals such as doctors, nurses, and therapists use scientific research to diagnose and treat symptoms and conditions. Examples of conventional medicine include pharmaceutical medications, physical rehabilitation, psychotherapy, radiation therapy, and surgery. Conventional medicine is based on modern science and evaluates the human body, its disorders, and medical treatments in purely biophysical or biochemical terms.

The main difference between holistic and conventional medicine is the approach to the patient and the treatment. Holistic medicine treats the patient as a whole person, not just a disease or a symptom; it uses a team approach involving the patient and the doctor and addresses all parts of a person's life using various healthcare practices.

Holistic medicine also emphasizes the responsibility of the patient for their health and well-being and the role of unconditional love and support as the most powerful healers. Conventional medicine treats the disease or the symptom, not the person, and uses a single or a few treatment methods, usually drugs, radiation, or surgery. Conventional medicine relies on the doctor's authority and the treatment's effectiveness rather than the patient's participation and empowerment.

The Principles and Benefits of Holistic Medicine for Allergic Rhinitis

Holistic medicine considers the whole person—body, mind, spirit, and emotions—to achieve optimal health and wellness. It uses various healthcare practices, from conventional to alternative, based on the belief that maintaining balance among these interconnected aspects is the primary goal. Some of the principles of holistic medicine are:

- All people have innate healing powers.
- The patient is a person, not a disease.

- Healing takes a team approach involving the patient and doctor and addresses all parts of a person's life using various healthcare practices.
- Treatment involves fixing the condition's cause, not just easing the symptoms.
- Prevention is preferable to treatment and is usually more cost-effective.
- The most cost-effective approach evokes the patient's innate healing capabilities.
- Illness is viewed as a manifestation of the dysfunction of the whole person, not as an isolated event.
- A major determinant of healing outcomes is the quality of the relationship established between physician and patient, in which patient autonomy is encouraged.
- The ideal physician-patient relationship considers the needs, desires, awareness, and insight of the patient as well as those of the physician.
- Physicians significantly influence patients through their example.

- Illness, pain, and the dying process can be learning opportunities for patients and physicians.

- Holistic physicians encourage patients to evoke the healing power of love, hope, humor, and enthusiasm and to release the toxic consequences of hostility, shame, greed, depression, and prolonged fear, anger, and grief.

- Unconditional love is life's most powerful medicine. Physicians strive to adopt an attitude of unconditional love for patients, themselves, and other practitioners.

- Optimal health is much more than the absence of sickness. It is the conscious pursuit of the highest qualities of the physical, environmental, mental, emotional, spiritual, and social aspects of the human experience.

Some of the benefits of holistic medicine for allergic rhinitis are:

- It can help identify and avoid the allergens that trigger your symptoms and reduce exposure.

- It can help relieve your symptoms and boost your immune system with natural remedies, such as herbs, supplements, essential oils, and homeopathy.

- It can help prevent and control inflammation and improve your respiratory health with a healthy lifestyle, such as diet, exercise, stress management, and sleep hygiene.

- It can help you cope with allergic rhinitis's emotional and social challenges and improve your mood and well-being.

- It can help treat the underlying causes of your condition, not just the symptoms, and address the whole person, not just the nose.

- It can help you take an active role in your health and well-being and empower you to make informed choices about your health care.

Holistic Methods Covered in This Book

This book will guide you through different holistic methods that can assist you in overcoming allergic rhinitis. This condition affects millions of people globally and can cause harm to both physical and mental health.

The holistic methods mentioned in this book are based on the principles of holistic medicine. Holistic medicine believes that the whole person, which includes the body, mind, spirit, and emotions, should be considered for optimal health and wellness. The holistic methods that will be covered in this book are:

- *Natural remedies,* such as herbs, supplements, essential oils, and homeopathy, can relieve symptoms and boost your immune system. You will discover these natural remedies' benefits, uses, and precautions and how to choose the best ones for your condition.
- *Lifestyle changes* like diet, exercise, stress management, and sleep hygiene can prevent and control inflammation and improve respiratory health. You will learn how to adopt a healthy and balanced lifestyle and how to avoid or minimize the factors that can worsen your condition, such as smoking, alcohol, pollution, and allergens.

- *Complementary therapies,* such as acupuncture, massage, yoga, meditation, and biofeedback, can enhance your well-being and support your healing process. You will learn how these therapies work, how to find a qualified practitioner, and how to integrate them into your daily routine.

How to Use Holistic Methods Safely and Effectively

Using holistic methods to treat allergic rhinitis can be a rewarding and empowering experience, but it also requires some caution and responsibility. Here are some general guidelines on how to use holistic methods safely and effectively:

- Consult your doctor before starting any holistic method, especially if you have a medical condition, are pregnant or breastfeeding, or are taking any medication. Some holistic methods may interact with your medication or worsen your condition, so it is important to get professional advice and supervision.

- Do your research before choosing a holistic method, and ensure you understand each method's benefits, risks, and limitations. Look for credible sources of information, such as scientific studies, reputable websites, or qualified practitioners. Avoid relying on anecdotal evidence, personal testimonials, or marketing claims that may be biased or misleading.

- Start slowly and gradually, and monitor your progress and reactions. Do not expect immediate or miraculous results, and do not overdo it. Some holistic methods may take time to show effects, and some may cause side effects or adverse reactions. Listen to your body and adjust your dosage, frequency, or intensity accordingly. If you experience any discomfort, pain, or worsening symptoms, stop the method and seek medical help.

- Be consistent and patient, and follow the instructions and recommendations of your holistic therapist or practitioner. Holistic methods are not quick fixes but long-term strategies requiring commitment and discipline. You need to follow the guidelines and stick to the plan to get the most out of your holistic method. Do not skip sessions, do not change the method without consulting your therapist or practitioner, and do not give up too soon.

- Combine different holistic methods to enhance their effects and address different aspects of your condition. Holistic therapy is not about choosing one method over another but instead integrating various methods to create a comprehensive and personalized treatment plan. For example, you can use natural remedies to relieve your symptoms, lifestyle changes to prevent inflammation, and complementary therapies to improve your well-being. By combining different holistic methods, you can achieve greater balance and harmony in your body, mind, and spirit.

Chapter 2

Natural Remedies for Allergic Rhinitis

Natural Remedies to Relieve Allergic Rhinitis Symptoms

Natural remedies are substances or practices derived from nature to treat or prevent a health condition. They are often considered complementary or alternatives to conventional medicine and may have fewer side effects or interactions.

However, they are not always scientifically proven or regulated and may vary in quality and effectiveness. Therefore, it is important to consult your doctor before using any natural remedy, especially if you have a medical condition, are pregnant or breastfeeding, or are taking any medication.

Some of the natural remedies that can help relieve allergic rhinitis symptoms are:

- Herbs, such as butterbur, stinging nettle, eyebright, and goldenseal, can reduce inflammation, histamine, and mucus production in the nasal passages. They can be taken as capsules, tablets, teas, or tinctures.
- Supplements, such as vitamin C, quercetin, bromelain, and omega-3 fatty acids, can boost the immune system, modulate the allergic response, and protect the mucous membranes from damage. They can be taken as pills, powders, or liquids.
- Essential oils, such as peppermint, eucalyptus, lavender, and lemon, can soothe nasal and sinus irritation, clear congestion, and fight infection. They can be inhaled, diffused, or applied topically with a carrier oil.

- Homeopathic remedies, such as Allium cepa, Arsenicum album, Euphrasia, and Nux vomica, can stimulate the body's natural healing ability and balance the energy flow. They can be taken as pellets, drops, or sprays.

How Each Natural Remedy Works and What Evidence Supports Its Use

Here is how each natural remedy works and what evidence supports its use for allergic rhinitis:

- **Herbs:** Herbs are plants that have medicinal properties and can be used to treat various health conditions. Some herbs that can help with allergic rhinitis are butterbur, stinging nettle, eyebright, and goldenseal. These herbs can reduce inflammation, histamine, and mucus production in the nasal passages and may have antihistamine, anti-inflammatory, or antibacterial effects. Some studies have shown that butterbur can be as effective as antihistamine drugs in reducing allergic rhinitis symptoms without causing drowsiness.

However, some herbs may also have side effects or interactions with other medications, so it is important to consult your doctor before using them.

- **Supplements:** Supplements are substances that provide extra nutrients or substances that may be lacking or insufficient in the diet. Some supplements that can help with allergic rhinitis are vitamin C, quercetin, bromelain, and omega-3 fatty acids. These supplements can boost the immune system, modulate the allergic response, and protect the mucous membranes from damage. Some studies have shown that vitamin C can lower histamine levels and improve nasal symptoms; quercetin can inhibit mast cell activation and inflammation; bromelain can enhance the absorption of quercetin and reduce swelling; and omega-3 fatty acids can reduce the production of inflammatory mediators. However, some supplements may also have side effects or interactions with other medications, so it is important to consult your doctor before using them.

- **Essential oils:** Essential oils are concentrated plant extracts with aromatic and therapeutic properties. Some essential oils that can help with allergic rhinitis are peppermint, eucalyptus, lavender, and lemon. These essential oils can soothe nasal and sinus irritation, clear congestion, and fight infection. Some studies have shown that peppermint oil can relax the smooth muscles and open the airways; eucalyptus oil can reduce inflammation and mucus secretion; lavender oil can have anti-inflammatory and antihistamine effects; and lemon oil can have antibacterial and antioxidant effects. However, some essential oils may also have side effects or interactions with other medications, so it is important to consult your doctor before using them.

- **Homeopathic remedies:** Homeopathic remedies are highly diluted substances prepared according to the principle of "like cures like," which means that a substance that causes symptoms in a healthy person can cure those symptoms in a sick person. Some homeopathic remedies that can help with allergic rhinitis are Allium cepa, Arsenicum album, Euphrasia, and Nux vomica. These remedies can stimulate the body's natural healing ability and balance the energy flow. Some studies have shown that homeopathic remedies can improve allergic rhinitis symptoms and quality of life and may have a similar effect as conventional antihistamines. However, some homeopathic remedies may also have side effects or interactions with other medications, so it is important to consult your doctor before using them.

How to Prepare and Use Each Natural Remedy for Allergic Rhinitis

Here is a demonstration of how to prepare and use each natural remedy for allergic rhinitis:

- **Herbs:** You can use herbs in various forms, such as capsules, tablets, teas, or tinctures. For example, to make an herbal tea, you can steep 1–2 teaspoons of dried herb or 2–4 teaspoons of fresh herb in a cup of boiling water for 10–15 minutes. Strain and drink 2–3 cups a day. To use a tincture, add 20–40 drops of the liquid extract to a glass of water or juice and drink 2-3 times daily. Follow the dosage and instructions on the label, or consult your doctor before using any herb.

- **Supplements:** You can take supplements as pills, powders, or liquids, depending on the form and availability. Follow the dosage and instructions on the label, or consult your doctor before using any supplement. For example, the recommended daily vitamin C intake for adults is 75–90 mg, but some studies suggest that higher doses of 1–2 g may benefit allergic rhinitis. Quercetin is usually taken in doses of 250–600 mg twice a day, 20 minutes before meals. Bromelain is usually taken in doses of 80–320 mg twice daily on an empty stomach.

Omega-3 fatty acids are usually taken in doses of 1–3 g per day with meals.

- **Essential oils:** You can use essential oils in various ways, such as inhalation, diffusion, or topical application. For inhalation, add 2–3 drops of essential oil to a bowl of hot water and inhale the steam for 5–10 minutes. For diffusion, you can use an aromatherapy diffuser or a humidifier to disperse the oil into the air. For topical application, you can dilute 2–3 drops of essential oil with a carrier oil, such as coconut, almond, or jojoba oil, and apply it to your chest, temples, or under your nose. Do a patch test before using any essential oil on your skin, and avoid contact with your eyes and mucous membranes.

- **Homeopathic remedies:** You can take homeopathic remedies as pellets, drops, or sprays, depending on the form and availability. Follow the dosage and instructions on the label, or consult your doctor before using any homeopathic remedy. For example, Allium cepa is usually taken in a 6C or 30C potency,

3–5 pellets every 15 minutes for acute symptoms or 3 times daily for chronic symptoms. Arsenicum album is usually taken in a 6C or 30C potency, 3–5 pellets every 2 hours for acute symptoms or twice daily for chronic symptoms. Euphrasia is usually taken in a 6C or 30C potency, 3–5 pellets every 4 hours for acute or chronic symptoms or once a day. Nux vomica is usually taken in a 6C or 30C potency, 3–5 pellets every hour for acute symptoms or 3 times daily for chronic symptoms.

Chapter 3

Lifestyle Changes for Allergic Rhinitis

Lifestyle Factors that Can Trigger or Worsen Allergic Rhinitis

Lifestyle factors are the aspects of your daily life that can affect your health and well-being. Some lifestyle factors can trigger or worsen allergic rhinitis. This condition causes inflammation and irritation in the nose, eyes, throat, and sinuses due to an allergic reaction to certain substances in the air, called allergens. Some of the lifestyle factors that can trigger or worsen allergic rhinitis are:

- **Diet:** Certain foods and drinks can cause or increase the symptoms of allergic rhinitis, such as sneezing, runny nose, and congestion. These include spicy foods, alcohol, dairy products, and foods that contain histamine, such as aged cheese, fermented foods, and cured meats. Some people may also have food allergies or intolerances that can trigger allergic rhinitis, such as gluten, eggs, nuts, or shellfish.

- **Stress:** Stress can affect the immune system and the nervous system, which can make you more sensitive to allergens and more prone to inflammation. Stress can also worsen the emotional and social impact of allergic rhinitis, such as anxiety, depression, and low self-esteem.

- **Environment:** The environment you live in or work in can expose you to various allergens or irritants that can trigger or worsen allergic rhinitis. These include pollen, dust mites, animal dander, mold, cockroaches, smoke, fumes, chemicals, and pollution. Weather changes, such as temperature, humidity, and wind, can also affect the levels and distribution of allergens in the air.

- **Habits:** Some habits or behaviors can increase your risk or severity of allergic rhinitis, such as smoking, drinking alcohol, using nasal decongestants, or picking your nose. Smoking can irritate the nasal and sinus passages, impair the cilia (tiny hairs) that clear the mucus, and reduce the effectiveness of medications. Drinking alcohol can dilate the blood vessels in the nose and cause swelling and congestion. Using nasal decongestants for more than three days can cause rebound congestion, which is when the nasal passages become more congested after the medication wears off. Picking your nose can damage the nasal lining and introduce bacteria or viruses that can cause infection.

How to Avoid Exposure to Allergens and Irritants that Cause Allergic Rhinitis

Allergic rhinitis is a condition that causes inflammation and irritation in the nose, eyes, throat, and sinuses due to an allergic reaction to certain substances in the air called allergens. Some of the common allergens that can trigger or worsen allergic rhinitis are pollen, dust mites, animal dander, mold, cockroaches, smoke, fumes, chemicals, and pollution. To avoid or reduce exposure to these allergens and irritants, you can follow these tips:

- **Identify your triggers.** The first step to avoiding or reducing exposure to allergens and irritants is to know what you are allergic to. You can do this by keeping a diary of your symptoms and activities or by getting an allergy test from your doctor.
- **Stay indoors when the pollen count is high.** Pollen is one of the most common triggers of allergic rhinitis, especially during spring, summer, and fall. You can check the pollen forecast in your area and plan your

outdoor activities accordingly. If you have to go outside, try to do it earlier in the day rather than later when the pollen levels are lower.

- **Keep your windows closed.** Another way to avoid or reduce exposure to pollen and other outdoor allergens and irritants is to keep your windows closed, especially during peak hours. You can also use air conditioning or air filters to clean the air in your home or car.

- **Clean your home regularly.** Dust mites, animal dander, mold, and cockroaches are some of the indoor allergens and irritants that can cause allergic rhinitis. To prevent or minimize their presence, you can clean your home regularly using a vacuum cleaner with a HEPA filter, a damp cloth, or a microfiber duster. You can also use allergen-proof covers for your pillows, mattresses, and box springs, and wash your bedding frequently in hot water.

- **Avoid smoking and secondhand smoke.** Smoke is a common irritant that can worsen allergic rhinitis symptoms, such as sneezing, runny nose, and congestion. If you smoke, try to quit or reduce your smoking. If you are exposed to secondhand smoke, try to avoid it or limit your exposure. You can also use a nasal saline spray or rinse to clear your nasal passages after exposure.

- **Wear a mask or carry portable oxygen.** If you have to be in an environment where you are exposed to allergens or irritants, such as a workplace, a public place, or a travel destination, you can wear a mask over your nose and mouth to filter the air you breathe. You can also carry portable oxygen if you have been prescribed oxygen therapy to help you breathe better.

How to Improve Diet and Nutrition to Boost Immunity and Reduce Inflammation

Diet and nutrition are important factors that can affect your immune system and inflammation levels. A healthy diet can help you prevent or fight infections, as well as reduce chronic inflammation that can lead to various diseases. Here are some recommendations on how to improve your diet and nutrition to boost your immunity and reduce inflammation:

- **Eat more fruits and vegetables.** Fruits and vegetables are rich in antioxidants, vitamins, minerals, and fiber that can help protect your cells from damage, support your immune system and lower inflammation. Aim for at least five servings of fruits and vegetables per day, and choose a variety of colors to get a range of phytochemicals.

- **Choose whole grains over refined grains.** Whole grains, such as oats, barley, quinoa, and brown rice, contain more nutrients and fiber than refined grains, such as white bread, pasta, and rice. Fiber can help feed the beneficial bacteria in your gut, which can modulate your immune system and reduce inflammation. Whole grains can also help lower your blood sugar and cholesterol levels, which can reduce your risk of diabetes and heart disease.

- **Include healthy fats in your diet.** Healthy fats, such as omega-3 fatty acids, monounsaturated fats, and polyunsaturated fats, can help reduce inflammation and improve your immune function. Omega-3 fatty acids are found in fatty fish, such as salmon, sardines, and mackerel, as well as in flaxseeds, chia seeds, and walnuts. Monounsaturated fats are found in olive oil, avocado, and nuts. Polyunsaturated fats are found in sunflower, corn, and soybean oils. Limit your intake of saturated fats, found in red meat, butter, and cheese, and avoid trans fats, found in processed foods, as they can increase inflammation and harm your health.

- **Add more spices and herbs to your meals.** Spices and herbs, such as turmeric, ginger, garlic, cinnamon, and rosemary, can add flavor and health benefits to your dishes. They contain bioactive compounds that can modulate your immune system, reduce inflammation, and fight infections. For example, turmeric contains curcumin, which can inhibit the production of inflammatory cytokines. Ginger contains gingerol, which can suppress the activation of inflammatory pathways. Garlic contains allicin, which can stimulate the activity of immune cells.

- **Drink enough water and limit alcohol.** Water is essential for your body's functions, including your immune system and inflammation. Water can help flush out toxins, transport nutrients, and oxygen, and regulate your body temperature. Aim for at least eight glasses of water per day, and more if you exercise or sweat a lot. Limit your intake of alcohol, as it can impair your immune system, increase inflammation, and damage your liver. If you drink alcohol, drink only in moderation, which means no more than one drink per day for women and two drinks per day for men.

How to Manage Stress and Emotions to Cope with Allergic Rhinitis

Stress and emotions can affect your immune system and inflammation levels, which can make you more sensitive to allergens and more prone to allergic rhinitis. Therefore, learning how to manage stress and emotions can help you cope with allergic rhinitis and improve your well-being. Here are some ways to manage stress and emotions to cope with allergic rhinitis:

- **Identify the sources of your stress and emotions.** The first step to managing stress and emotions is to recognize what triggers them and how they affect you. You can do this by keeping a journal of your thoughts, feelings, and reactions or by talking to someone you trust, such as a friend, family member, or therapist.

- **Practice relaxation techniques.** Relaxation techniques can help you calm your mind and body and reduce the effects of stress and emotions on your immune system and inflammation. Some relaxation techniques include deep breathing, meditation, yoga, progressive muscle relaxation, and guided imagery. You can practice these techniques daily or whenever you feel stressed or emotional.

- **Work out as a part of your daily routine.** Physical activity can help you release stress and emotions and improve your mood and health. Exercise can also help you breathe better as it releases the hormone epinephrine, which acts as a natural decongestant and can open your airways. You can choose an activity that you enjoy, such as walking, jogging, cycling, swimming, or dancing, and do it for at least 30 minutes three times a week.

- **Seek social support.** Social support can help you cope with stress and emotions and provide you with comfort, advice, and encouragement. You can seek social support from people who understand your condition and respect your feelings, such as your family, friends, support groups, or online communities. You can also join activities or hobbies that can help you connect with others and have fun, such as volunteering, joining a club, or taking a class.

- **Challenge negative thoughts.** Negative thoughts can increase your stress and emotions and make you feel worse about your condition. You can challenge negative thoughts by identifying them, questioning their validity, and replacing them with more positive and realistic ones. For example, if you think, "I cannot do anything because of my allergies," you can challenge it by asking yourself, "Is this true? What evidence do I have? What can I do to improve my situation?" and replace it with "I can do many things despite my allergies, and I can find ways to manage my symptoms and enjoy my life."

Creating a Healthy and Comfortable Environment for Nose and Sinuses

Creating a healthy and comfortable environment for the nose and sinuses can help you prevent or relieve allergic rhinitis symptoms such as sneezing, runny nose, and congestion. Here are some tips on how to create a healthy and comfortable environment for the nose and sinuses:

- Use a humidifier or a vaporizer to add moisture to the air, especially in dry or cold weather. This can help keep the nasal and sinus passages moist and prevent them from drying out and becoming irritated. You can also use a saline nasal spray or rinse to hydrate and cleanse your nose and sinuses.
- Avoid exposure to allergens and irritants that can trigger or worsen allergic rhinitis, such as pollen, dust mites, animal dander, mold, smoke, fumes, chemicals, and pollution. You can do this by keeping your windows closed, using air filters or purifiers, cleaning your home regularly, wearing a mask, and avoiding smoking or secondhand smoke.
- Maintain a comfortable temperature and humidity level in your home and workplace. Extreme heat or cold or sudden changes in temperature or humidity can irritate the nasal and sinus membranes and cause swelling and

congestion. You can use a thermostat or a hygrometer to monitor and adjust the temperature and humidity levels in your environment.

- Take a hot shower or inhale steam from a bowl of hot water to help ease congestion and swelling in the nose and sinuses. You can also add a few drops of essential oils, such as peppermint, eucalyptus, lavender, or lemon, to the water to enhance the effect. Be careful not to burn yourself with the hot water or steam.

- Use a warm compress or a heating pad to apply gentle heat to your face, especially around your nose, cheeks, and forehead. This can help soothe the pain and pressure caused by inflammation and infection in the sinuses. You can also massage your face gently to stimulate blood circulation and drainage.

Chapter 4

Complementary Therapies for Allergic Rhinitis

Complementary Therapies That Help Treat Allergic Rhinitis

Complementary therapies are healthcare practices that are used along with conventional medicine to enhance the overall well-being of the patient. They are often based on traditional, holistic, or natural approaches to healing and may have physical, mental, emotional, or spiritual benefits.

Some of the complementary therapies that can help treat allergic rhinitis, a condition that causes inflammation and irritation in the nose, eyes, throat, and sinuses due to an allergic reaction to certain substances in the air, are:

- **Acupuncture:** Acupuncture is a technique that involves inserting thin needles into specific points on the body to stimulate the flow of energy and restore balance. Acupuncture can help reduce allergic rhinitis symptoms, such as sneezing, runny nose, and congestion, by modulating the immune system, reducing inflammation, and relieving stress.

- **Yoga:** Yoga is a practice that combines physical postures, breathing exercises, and meditation to promote health and harmony. Yoga can help improve allergic rhinitis symptoms, such as nasal obstruction, itching, and discharge, by enhancing respiratory function, strengthening the immune system, and calming the mind.

- **Meditation:** Meditation is a technique that involves focusing attention on a single object, thought, or sensation or simply being aware of the present moment to achieve a state of relaxation and awareness. Meditation can help alleviate allergic rhinitis symptoms, such as sneezing, runny nose, and congestion, by reducing stress, improving mood, and regulating the nervous system.

- **Massage:** Massage is a therapy that involves applying pressure, movement, or vibration to the soft tissues of the body, such as muscles, tendons, and ligaments, to improve circulation, relieve tension, and promote healing. Massage can help ease allergic rhinitis symptoms, such as headache, facial pain, and pressure, by stimulating lymphatic drainage, increasing blood flow, and relaxing the muscles.

How to Practice or Receive Complementary Therapy

Here is a demonstration of how to practice or receive each complementary therapy for allergic rhinitis:

- **Acupuncture:** To receive acupuncture, you need to find a qualified and licensed acupuncturist who has experience treating allergic rhinitis. You can search for an acupuncturist near you on the National Certification Commission for Acupuncture and Oriental Medicine website. You can also ask your doctor for a referral or recommendation. During an acupuncture session, the acupuncturist will insert thin needles into specific points on your body, usually on your face, head, neck, arms, or legs. The needles will stay in place for 15 to 30 minutes while you relax on a table. You may feel a slight sensation of tingling, warmth, or pressure, but it should not be painful. The acupuncturist may also use other techniques, such as moxibustion, cupping, or electroacupuncture, to enhance the effect. The number and frequency of sessions will depend on your condition and response, but typically, you will need several sessions over a few weeks or months.

- **Yoga:** To practice yoga, you need to find a suitable style, level, and instructor that suits your needs and preferences. You can search for a yoga class near you on the Yoga Alliance website, or you can practice at home with online videos or apps. You can also ask your doctor for a recommendation or a referral to a yoga therapist. During a yoga session, you will perform a series of physical postures, breathing exercises, and meditation guided by the instructor. You will need comfortable clothing, a yoga mat, and possibly some props, such as blocks, straps, or blankets. Practice yoga at least once a week, preferably more often, for at least 20 to 30 minutes per session. You should also practice yoga on an empty stomach or at least two hours after a meal. You should avoid yoga poses that put pressure on your face, head, or sinuses, such as headstands, forward bends, or inversions, unless instructed otherwise by your instructor.

- **Meditation:** To practice meditation, you need to find a quiet and comfortable place where you can sit or lie down without distractions. You can use a cushion, a chair, or a bed to support your posture. You can also use a timer, a music player, or an app to help you meditate. You can choose from different types of meditation, such as mindfulness, mantras, or guided imagery, depending on your preference and goal. During a meditation session, you will focus your attention on a single object, thought, or sensation or be aware of the present moment and let go of any thoughts or feelings that arise. You will breathe deeply and slowly, and you will relax your body and mind. Practice meditation at least once a day, preferably more often, for at least 10 to 20 minutes per session. You can also practice meditation whenever you feel stressed or emotional, or before or after other activities, such as yoga or acupuncture.

- **Massage:** To receive a massage, you need to find a qualified and licensed massage therapist who has experience treating allergic rhinitis. You can search for a massage therapist near you on the American Massage Therapy Association website, or you can ask your doctor for a referral or recommendation. During a massage session, the massage therapist will apply pressure, movement, or vibration to the soft tissues of your body, such as your muscles, tendons, and ligaments. The massage therapist will focus on your face, head, neck, and shoulders and may also massage other parts of your body, depending on your needs and preferences. You will need to undress to your level of comfort and lie on a table covered with a sheet or a towel. You may also use oil, lotion, or aromatherapy to enhance the effect. The massage session will last for 30 to 60 minutes, and you will feel relaxed and refreshed afterward. The number and frequency of sessions will depend on your condition and response, but typically, you will need one or two sessions per week for a few weeks or months.

The Advantages and Limitations of Complementary Therapy

Each complementary therapy for allergic rhinitis has its advantages and limitations, depending on the evidence, safety, availability, and cost of the therapy. Here are the pros and cons of each therapy:

- **Acupuncture:** Acupuncture is a technique that involves inserting thin needles into specific points on the body to stimulate the flow of energy and restore balance. Acupuncture can help reduce allergic rhinitis symptoms, such as sneezing, runny nose, and congestion, by modulating the immune system, reducing inflammation, and relieving stress. The advantages of acupuncture are that it is a non-invasive, natural, and holistic therapy that can address the root cause of the condition, not just the symptoms. It can also improve the overall well-being and quality of life of the patient. The limitations of acupuncture are that it may not be effective for everyone, it may require multiple sessions and maintenance treatments, and it may have some side effects or risks, such as bleeding, bruising, infection, or nerve damage. It may also be difficult to find a qualified and licensed acupuncturist, and it may not be covered by insurance.

- **Yoga:** Yoga is a practice that combines physical postures, breathing exercises, and meditation to promote health and harmony. Yoga can help improve allergic rhinitis symptoms, such as nasal obstruction, itching, and discharge, by enhancing respiratory function, strengthening the immune system, and calming the mind. The advantages of yoga are that it is a low-cost, accessible, and enjoyable therapy that can benefit the physical, mental, emotional, and spiritual aspects of the patient. It can also prevent or reduce the risk of other chronic diseases, such as diabetes, hypertension, and obesity. The limitations of yoga are that it may not be suitable for everyone, especially those with certain medical conditions, injuries, or disabilities. It may also require guidance and supervision from a trained instructor, and it may take time and practice to achieve the desired results.

- **Meditation:** Meditation is a technique that involves focusing attention on a single object, thought, or sensation or simply being aware of the present moment to achieve a state of relaxation and awareness. Meditation can help alleviate allergic rhinitis symptoms, such as sneezing, runny nose, and congestion, by reducing stress, improving mood, and regulating the nervous system. The advantages of meditation are that it is a simple, free, and flexible therapy that can be practiced anywhere and anytime and that can enhance the cognitive, emotional, and social skills of the patient. It can also improve the coping and resilience of the patient and reduce the need for medication. The limitations of meditation are that it may be challenging for everyone, especially those who need help with concentrating, relaxing, or sitting still. It may also require patience and perseverance, and it may not be sufficient to treat severe or persistent symptoms.

- **Massage:** Massage is a therapy that involves applying pressure, movement, or vibration to the soft tissues of the body, such as muscles, tendons, and ligaments, to improve circulation, relieve tension, and promote healing. Massage can help ease allergic rhinitis symptoms, such as headache, facial pain, and pressure, by stimulating lymphatic drainage, increasing blood flow, and relaxing the muscles. The advantages of massage are that it is a relaxing, soothing, and pleasurable therapy that can reduce the pain and discomfort associated with allergic rhinitis and improve nasal patency and sinus function. The limitations of massage are that it may be expensive, time-consuming, and inconvenient and that it may have some side effects or contraindications, such as bruising, swelling, infection, or aggravation of existing conditions. Additionally, it could not be easy to locate a licensed and qualified massage therapist, and insurance might not cover it.

Chapter 5

Prevention and Maintenance for Allergic Rhinitis

Tips to Prevent or Reduce the Frequency and Severity of Allergic Rhinitis Episodes

Allergic rhinitis is a condition that causes inflammation and irritation in the nose, eyes, throat, and sinuses due to an allergic reaction to certain substances in the air called allergens. Allergic rhinitis can affect your quality of life, productivity, and well-being and can increase your risk of developing other conditions, such as sinusitis, asthma, or ear infections.

Therefore, it is important to prevent or reduce the frequency and severity of allergic rhinitis episodes by following these strategies and tips:

- Avoid or reduce exposure to allergens and irritants that can trigger or worsen allergic rhinitis, such as pollen, dust mites, animal dander, mold, smoke, fumes, chemicals, and pollution. You can do this by keeping your windows closed, using air filters or purifiers, cleaning your home regularly, wearing a mask, and avoiding smoking or secondhand smoke.

- Improve your diet and nutrition to boost your immunity and reduce inflammation. You can do this by eating more fruits and vegetables, choosing whole grains over refined grains, including healthy fats in your diet, adding more spices and herbs to your meals, drinking enough water, and limiting alcohol.

- Manage your stress and emotions to cope with allergic rhinitis. You can do this by identifying the sources of your stress and emotions, practicing relaxation techniques, working out as a part of your daily routine, seeking social support, and challenging negative thoughts.

- Create a healthy and comfortable environment for your nose and sinuses. You can do this by using a humidifier or vaporizer to add moisture to the air, taking a hot shower or inhaling steam to ease congestion and swelling, using a warm compress or a heating pad to soothe pain and pressure, and using a saline nasal spray or rinse to hydrate and cleanse your nose and sinuses.

- Use complementary therapies to enhance your well-being and support your healing process. You can do this by practicing or receiving acupuncture, yoga, meditation, or massage, which can help modulate your immune system, reduce inflammation, and relieve stress.

- Follow your doctor's advice and treatment plan for allergic rhinitis. You can accomplish this by taking your doctor-prescribed medications, such as antihistamines, decongestants, corticosteroids, or leukotriene modifiers, as directed and only when necessary. You can also ask your doctor about other options, such as immunotherapy, which can help desensitize your immune system to allergens and reduce your symptoms in the long term.

How to Monitor, Track Symptoms and Triggers Over Time

Monitoring and tracking your symptoms and triggers over time can help you understand your condition better, identify patterns and trends, and manage your allergic rhinitis more effectively. Here are some ways to monitor and track your symptoms and triggers over time:

- Keep a diary or a journal of your symptoms and triggers. You can use a notebook, a calendar, an app, or a website to record your symptoms and triggers every day. You can also rate the severity of your symptoms and their impact on your quality of life using a scale from 0 to 10. You can include information such as the date, time, duration, location, weather, activities, foods, medications, and treatments related to your symptoms and triggers.

- Review your diary or journal regularly. You can look for patterns and trends in your symptoms and triggers, such as seasonal variations, environmental factors, or lifestyle habits. You can also compare your symptoms and triggers with the pollen forecast in your area or with the results of your allergy test if you have one. You can use charts, graphs, or tables to visualize your data and make it easier to understand.

- Share your diary or journal with your doctor or allergist. You can use your diary or journal as a tool to communicate with your doctor or allergist about your condition. You can show them your symptoms and triggers and how they affect your well-being. You can also ask them for feedback, advice, or recommendations on how to prevent or reduce your symptoms and triggers and how to adjust your treatment plan accordingly.

Adjusting the Holistic Treatment Plan According to Individual Needs and Goals

A holistic treatment plan for allergic rhinitis is a comprehensive and personalized approach that aims to address the physical, mental, emotional, and spiritual aspects of the condition. A holistic treatment plan can include various elements, such as natural remedies, lifestyle changes, and complementary therapies, that can help prevent, reduce, or treat the symptoms and the underlying causes of allergic rhinitis. However, a holistic treatment plan is not a one-size-fits-all solution, and it may need to be adjusted according to the individual needs and goals of each patient. Here are some factors to consider when adjusting the holistic treatment plan for allergic rhinitis:

- The severity and frequency of the symptoms. The holistic treatment plan should be tailored to the severity of allergic rhinitis symptoms, which include sneezing, runny nose, congestion, itching, and headaches. For mild or intermittent symptoms, the holistic treatment plan may focus more on prevention and natural remedies, such as avoiding allergens, improving diet and nutrition, and using herbs, supplements, or essential oils. For moderate or persistent symptoms, the holistic treatment plan may include more medication and complementary therapies, such as antihistamines, decongestants, corticosteroids, acupuncture, yoga, or massage.

- The type and source of the allergens. The holistic treatment plan should be based on the specific allergens that trigger or worsen allergic rhinitis, such as pollen, dust mites, animal dander, mold, or smoke. The type and source of the allergens can be identified by keeping a diary of the symptoms and triggers or by getting an allergy test from a doctor or an allergist. Depending on the type and source of the allergens, the holistic treatment plan may involve different strategies to avoid or reduce exposure, such as staying indoors, using air filters, cleaning the home, or wearing a mask. The holistic treatment plan may also consider the possibility of immunotherapy, which is a treatment that can desensitize the immune system to allergens and reduce symptoms in the long term.

- The personal preferences and values of the patient. The holistic treatment plan should respect and accommodate the personal preferences and values of the patient, such as their beliefs, expectations, goals, and motivations. The holistic treatment plan should be based on a shared decision-making process between the patient and the healthcare provider and should involve the patient's active participation and consent. The holistic treatment plan should also consider the patient's preferences and values regarding the different elements of the plan, such as the type, dosage, frequency, and duration of the natural remedies, lifestyle changes, and complementary therapies. The holistic treatment plan should also address any concerns or barriers that the patient may have, such as cost, availability, accessibility, safety, or effectiveness of the elements of the plan.

Communicating and Collaborating with Healthcare Provider and Support Network

Communication and collaboration are essential skills for managing allergic rhinitis. This condition causes inflammation and irritation in the nose, eyes, throat, and sinuses due to an allergic reaction to certain substances in the air, called allergens. By communicating and collaborating with your healthcare provider and support network, you can improve your health outcomes, well-being, and quality of life. Here are some tips on how to communicate and collaborate with your healthcare provider and support network:

- **With your healthcare provider:** Your healthcare provider is your partner in your holistic treatment plan, which may include natural remedies, lifestyle changes, complementary therapies, and medication. You should communicate openly and honestly with your healthcare provider about your symptoms, triggers, preferences, values, and goals. You should also ask questions, seek clarification, and express any concerns or doubts you may have about your condition or treatment. You should collaborate with your healthcare provider by following their advice and instructions, taking your medication as prescribed, and reporting any changes or problems you may experience. You should also share your diary or journal of your symptoms and triggers and any information or evidence you may have about the natural remedies, lifestyle changes, or complementary therapies you are using or interested in.

- **With your support network:** Your support network may include your family, friends, support groups, or online communities. They can provide you with comfort, advice, encouragement, and practical help. You should communicate clearly and respectfully with your support network about your condition, your needs, and your boundaries. You should also listen to their feedback, suggestions, and experiences and appreciate their support and involvement. You should collaborate with your support network by asking for help when you need it, accepting their assistance and generosity, and reciprocating their kindness and care. You should also join activities or hobbies that can help you connect with others and have fun, such as volunteering, joining a club, or taking a class.

Conclusion

This book has provided you with a holistic approach to managing allergic rhinitis, a condition that causes inflammation and irritation in the nose, eyes, throat, and sinuses due to an allergic reaction to certain substances in the air, called allergens. Here are some of the main takeaways and lessons from this book:

- Allergic rhinitis can affect your quality of life, productivity, and well-being and can increase your risk of developing other conditions, such as sinusitis, asthma, or ear infections. Therefore, it is important to prevent or reduce the frequency and severity of allergic rhinitis episodes by following a holistic treatment plan that addresses the physical, mental, emotional, and spiritual aspects of the condition.

- A holistic treatment plan for allergic rhinitis can include various elements, such as natural remedies, lifestyle changes, and complementary therapies, that can help prevent, reduce, or treat the symptoms and the underlying causes of allergic rhinitis. Some of the natural remedies are herbs, supplements, essential oils, and homeopathic remedies. Some of the lifestyle changes are diet and nutrition, stress and emotions, and environment and habits. Some of the complementary therapies are acupuncture, yoga, meditation, and massage.

- A holistic treatment plan for allergic rhinitis is not a one-size-fits-all solution, and it may need to be adjusted according to the individual needs and goals of each patient. Some of the factors to consider when adjusting the holistic treatment plan are the severity and frequency of the symptoms, the type and source of the allergens, and the personal preferences and values of the patient.

- Communication and collaboration are essential skills for managing allergic rhinitis. By communicating and collaborating with your healthcare provider and support network, you can improve your health outcomes, well-being, and quality of life. You should communicate openly and honestly with your healthcare provider about your symptoms, triggers, preferences, values, and goals. You should also ask questions, seek clarification, and express any concerns or doubts you may have about your condition or treatment.

You should collaborate with your healthcare provider by following their advice and instructions, taking your medication as prescribed, and reporting any changes or problems you may experience. You should also share your diary or journal of your symptoms and triggers and any information or evidence you may have about the natural remedies, lifestyle changes, or complementary therapies you are using or interested in. You should communicate clearly and respectfully with your support network about your condition, your needs, and your boundaries.

You should also listen to their feedback, suggestions, and experiences and appreciate their support and involvement. You should collaborate with your support network by asking for help when you need it, accepting their assistance and generosity, and reciprocating their kindness and care. You should also join activities or hobbies that can help you connect with others and have fun, such as volunteering, joining a club, or taking a class.

The Challenges and Opportunities for Patients Living with Allergic Rhinitis

Living with allergic rhinitis can be challenging but also rewarding. Allergic rhinitis is a condition that causes inflammation and irritation in the nose, eyes, throat, and sinuses due to an allergic reaction to certain substances in the air, called allergens.

Allergic rhinitis can affect your quality of life, productivity, and well-being and can increase your risk of developing other conditions, such as sinusitis, asthma, or ear infections. However, allergic rhinitis can also be an opportunity to learn more about yourself, your health, and your environment and to adopt a holistic approach to managing your condition and enhancing your well-being.

Some of the challenges of living with allergic rhinitis are:

- Dealing with the symptoms, such as sneezing, runny nose, congestion, itching, and headache, which can be uncomfortable, annoying, and disruptive.
- Avoiding or reducing exposure to allergens and irritants that can trigger or worsen allergic rhinitis, such as pollen, dust mites, animal dander, mold, smoke, fumes, chemicals, and pollution, which can be difficult, inconvenient, or costly,
- Finding the right treatment plan that works for you, which may include natural remedies,

lifestyle changes, complementary therapies, and medication, may vary depending on the severity and frequency of your symptoms, the type and source of your allergens, and your personal preferences and values.

- Communicating and collaborating with your healthcare provider and support network may involve sharing your symptoms, triggers, preferences, values, and goals, asking questions, seeking clarification, expressing concerns or doubts, following advice and instructions, reporting changes or problems, and appreciating support and involvement.

- Managing your stress and emotions, which can affect your immune system and inflammation levels, can be influenced by your condition, your symptoms, your triggers, your treatment, and your environment.

Some of the opportunities for living with allergic rhinitis are:

- Learning more about your condition, your symptoms, your triggers, your treatment, and your well-being can help you understand your condition better, identify patterns and trends, and manage your allergic rhinitis more effectively.

- Improving your diet and nutrition, which can help boost your immunity and reduce inflammation, can benefit your physical, mental, emotional, and spiritual health.

- Practicing relaxation techniques such as deep breathing, meditation, yoga, progressive muscle relaxation, and guided imagery can help calm your mind and body and reduce the effects of stress and emotions on your immune system and inflammation.

- Creating a healthy and comfortable environment for your nose and sinuses can help prevent or relieve allergic rhinitis symptoms and improve your nasal and sinus health and function.

- Using complementary therapies, such as acupuncture, yoga, meditation, or massage, which can help modulate your immune system, reduce inflammation, and relieve stress, can enhance your well-being and support your healing process.

Motivation to Help Readers Overcome Allergic Rhinitis Holistically and Effectively

You have just finished reading a book that has provided you with a holistic approach to managing allergic rhinitis, a condition that causes inflammation and irritation in the nose, eyes, throat, and sinuses due to an allergic reaction to certain substances in the air, called allergens.

You have learned about the causes, symptoms, and complications of allergic rhinitis and how to prevent or reduce them by using natural remedies, lifestyle changes, and complementary therapies. You have also learned how to adjust your holistic treatment plan according to your individual needs and goals and how to communicate and collaborate with your healthcare provider and support network.

Now, you may be wondering how to put this knowledge into practice and how to overcome allergic rhinitis holistically and effectively. You may be feeling overwhelmed, confused, or doubtful about your condition or treatment. You may be facing challenges, barriers, or setbacks in your journey to a happier and healthier life. You may be looking for some motivation and inspiration to keep going and achieve your desired results.

If that is the case, then I am here to help you. I am your assistant, and I am here to support you, guide you, and cheer you on. I am here to remind you of your strengths, your potential, and your possibilities. I am here to empower you, encourage you, and celebrate you. Here are some motivational and inspirational messages that I hope will help you overcome allergic rhinitis holistically and effectively:

- You are not alone. You are not the only one who suffers from allergic rhinitis, and you are not the only one who seeks a holistic solution. Millions of people around the world share your condition and your vision and are willing to support you and learn from you. You can connect with them through your family, friends, support groups, or online communities and exchange your experiences, insights, and tips. You can also rely on your healthcare provider and your support network, who are there to help you and care for you. You are part of a larger community that understands you and values you.

- You are in control. You are the one who knows your condition best, and you are the one who decides your treatment plan. You have the power and the responsibility to choose what works for you and to make changes when needed. You have the freedom and flexibility to explore different options and find your balance. You have the ability and the opportunity to influence your health and well-being and to create your reality.

- You are capable. You have the skills and resources to manage your allergic rhinitis and improve your quality of life. You have the knowledge and the wisdom to understand your condition, your symptoms, and your triggers, and to prevent or reduce them. You have the tools and the techniques to use natural remedies, lifestyle changes, and complementary therapies and to benefit from them. You have the strategies and tips to monitor and track your symptoms and triggers and to adjust your treatment plan accordingly. You have the communication and collaboration skills to work with your healthcare provider and support network and to receive their feedback and support.

- You are resilient. You have the strength and the courage to face your challenges, overcome your barriers, and cope with your setbacks. You have the perseverance and the patience to keep trying, keep learning, and keep improving. You have the optimism and hope to see the positive aspects of your condition and to appreciate the opportunities it offers. You have the gratitude and the joy to celebrate your achievements and to acknowledge your progress.

- You are amazing. You are a unique and wonderful person who has so much to offer the world. You are more than your condition, and you are not defined by your symptoms. You have your personality, interests, talents, and passions, and you can pursue them and express them. You have your dreams, goals, and aspirations, and you can achieve them and fulfill them. You have your value, worth, and dignity, and you can respect and honor them.

I pray these messages motivate and inspire you to overcome allergic rhinitis holistically and effectively. I hope you feel confident, empowered, and inspired to take action and make a difference. I hope you realize how amazing you are and how much potential you have.

I hope this book has helped you learn more about allergic rhinitis and how to manage it holistically. I hope you have found some useful tips and strategies that can improve your health and well-being. I hope you have enjoyed reading this book and have gained some valuable insights and knowledge. Thank you for choosing this book and for trusting me as your assistant. I wish you all the best in your journey to a happier and healthier life.

References and Resources

Here are some references and resources that you may find helpful for learning more about allergic rhinitis and how to manage it holistically and effectively:

Scientific Studies and Research Referenced:

- Allergic Rhinitis: A Clinical and Pathophysiological Overview - This article provides a comprehensive review of the epidemiology, diagnosis, and treatment of allergic rhinitis, as well as the current understanding of its pathophysiology and immunology.

- Allergic rhinitis - Allergy, Asthma & Clinical Immunology - This article summarizes the key aspects of allergic rhinitis, including its causes, symptoms, complications, diagnosis, and management, based on the Canadian guidelines published in 2007.

- Special Issue "Recent Advances in Allergic Rhinitis" - MDPI - This is a collection of articles that cover various topics related to allergic rhinitis, such as epidemiology, genetics, biomarkers, comorbidities, diagnosis, treatment, and prevention.

- Epidemiology, Prevention and Clinical Treatment of Allergic Rhinitis ... - This is a book chapter that provides an overview of the epidemiology, prevention, and clinical treatment of allergic rhinitis, with a focus on the role of allergen immunotherapy.

Recommended Books and Publications:

- Allergic Rhinitis: Rapid Evidence Review | AAFP - This is a rapid evidence review that highlights the current literature and research on the diagnosis and treatment of allergic rhinitis, based on the guidelines from the International Consensus Statement on Allergy and Rhinology (ICAR) 2023.

- Allergic Rhinitis | IntechOpen - This is a book that provides a holistic approach to managing allergic rhinitis, covering the causes, symptoms, and complications of the condition, as well as the natural remedies, lifestyle changes, and complementary therapies that can help prevent, reduce, or treat the symptoms and the underlying causes of allergic rhinitis.

- A Synopsis of Guidance for Allergic Rhinitis Diagnosis and Management ... - This is a synopsis of the ICAR 2023 guidelines for allergic rhinitis diagnosis and management, which provide evidence-based recommendations for health professionals on a worldwide basis.

- Global Atlas of Allergic Rhinitis and Chronic Rhinosinusitis - This is a publication that provides a global overview of allergic rhinitis and chronic rhinosinusitis, including the epidemiology, burden, diagnosis, treatment, and prevention of these conditions, as well as the current challenges and future perspectives.

Useful Organizations, Websites, and Support Groups:

- Rhinitis: Global Overview | World Allergy Organization - This is a website that provides information and resources about rhinitis, including its definition, classification, diagnosis, management, and complications, as well as the links between rhinitis and asthma.
- A List of Allergy Support Organizations and Resources - Allergies.net - This is a website that provides a list of allergy support organizations and resources, such as magazines, networks, associations, foundations, and initiatives, that can help people living with allergies and those who want to learn more about them.
- AAFA's Asthma and Allergy Communities | AAFA.org - This is a website that provides online communities and local support groups for patients with asthma and allergies, where they can connect with others, share their experiences, and get support and advice.